25 Paleo Asian Recipes

By Tina Fere

Table of Contents

Introduction

I want to thank and congratulate you for downloading the book *"25 Paleo Asian Recipes"*.

The Paleo Diet is considered as the world's healthiest diet because it makes use of the food products that our ancestors used to eat in order to promote optimal health. If you try the Paleo Diet, you'll be protected against diabetes, heart diseases, auto-immune diseases and you'll get to lose weight in the natural way, too!

The Paleo Diet Food List consists of:

• Fish

• Seafood

• Grass-Produced Meat

• Nuts and Seeds

• Eggs

• Fresh, Organic Fruits and Vegetables

• Healthy Oils, such as walnut, olive, flaxseed, avocado, macadamia and coconut

With the help of this book, you will learn to create amazing Asian-Inspired Paleo Recipes that will surely make you feel more delighted to it. Asian Cuisine is flavorful and tasty and that's why it's good to put a twist on those Paleo dishes with Asian flavors.

If eating healthy and nutritious dishes are your thing, it's time for you to start reading this book!

Once again, thank you and good luck!

Chapter 1: Oh so Awesome Breakfast Meals

Breakfast is the most important meal of the day. Without eating a proper breakfast meal, you would certainly feel tired and spent even if you haven't done enough for the day. To prevent that from happening, you have to try these awesome dishes below!

1. Sunshiny Omelet

(Makes 2 servings)

(Start your day right with an amazing and warm omelet that's sure to make you think of the sun and all warm, fuzzy things!)

Ingredients:

- 1 tsp olive oil

- 2 large range-free eggs, scrambled

- 2 green onions, diced

- 2 small organic tomatoes

- 1 cup fresh spinach leaves

- ½ fresh avocado, sliced into small pieces

Directions:

- In a non-stick pan, heat some oil and sauté the onions until they are tender.

• Add the eggs and cook for 2 minutes in low heat before adding the rest of the ingredients.

• Fold the omelet and flip it. Cook until eggs are well-done.

• Serve and enjoy!

Health Benefits/Fun Facts:

• Did you know that a man named Howard Helmer has 3 Guinness World Records for making 427 omelets in just 30 minutes? Wow!

• Range-free eggs are great because hens that stay in just one canopy lay them. This way you can be sure that they're clean and healthy.

• Avocados are quite beneficial because they are a good source of fats (the healthy kind), and good sources of dietary fiber, too! Because of this, cholesterol production in the body can be reduced and other diseases such as heart problems and strokes can be prevented, too!

• Green Onions are better than their contemporaries because they are good for bone health.

• Green Onions are also full of Vitamin A that is essential for great eye health and can also protect the immune system and the heart from various diseases—and that's mainly the reason why you shouldn't take green onions for granted!

2. Bacon and Avocado Omelet

(Makes 2 servings)

Ingredients:

- 1 avocado

- 4 bacon slices

- 1 Tbsp fresh cilantro, minced

- 1 Tbsp red onion, minced

- 4 eggs

- A dash of hot sauce

Directions:

- Cook the bacon until it is crispy. While the bacon is cooking, crack the avocado open. Remove the pit, and then scoop the flesh out and place it in a bowl. Mash until it reaches your desired consistency.

- Add cilantro and onions to the avocado mash. Drain all the oil from the bacon once it is done cooking. Stir all of the ingredients together.

- Make the omelet by folding the ingredients in and make sure to use the avocado mixture that you have just made.

- Serve omelets with hot sauce, if desired.

Health Benefits/Fun Facts:

- Contrary to popular belief, bacon is actually healthy because it contains essential vitamins and minerals such as Vitamin B1, Vitamin B3, Iron, Protein and Magnesium. It also builds up your stamina and helps the brain become smarter and more alert!

• Did you know? Mayonnaise made from bacon is actually considered Vegetarian, and September 3rd is actually International Bacon Day!

• Eggs are good for you because they lower the risk of developing cataracts. They also contain high amounts of protein and because of that, it is said that eating an egg a day may prevent macular degeneration and will protect you against various diseases!

3. Healthy Chicken Pad Thai

(Makes 4 servings)

Ingredients:

• 2 eggs, beaten lightly

• 1 small spaghetti squash, roasted or cooked

• 1 large chicken breast, cut into small strips

• 2 to 3 Tbsp avocado oil

• 2 cups mushrooms, sliced thinly

• 1 cup scallions, sliced thinly

• **For the sauce:** ¼ cup apple cider vinegar

• ¼ cup coconut aminos

• Garlic powder, to taste

• Sriracha, to taste

• **For garnish:** bean sprouts

• Fresh cilantro

• Lime wedges

Directions:

• Make the sauce first. To do this, mix garlic powder, sriracha, coconut aminos and apple cider vinegar altogether in a bowl then simmer and stir once in a while. Season to taste.

• Heat a non-stick pan until it starts to smoke a bit, and then add the avocado oil and spread it around the pan. Toss in the chicken slices, scallions and mushrooms. Cook for around 3 to 5 minutes or until heated through and make sure to stir frequently.

• Mix the spaghetti squash in then cook and stir for another minute or two or until it is cooked through. Add the eggs and stir until well-cooked.

• Add the sauce then go on and stir again. Cook for another 3 to 5 minutes then garnish with your choice of toppings before serving.

• Enjoy!

Health Benefits/Fun Facts:

• Pad-Thai is usually served in the streets and eateries of Thailand. It basically translates to "Fried Thai Style" made with tofu and sometimes served with Tamarind Pulp or Fish Sauce.

• Squash is usually made into spaghetti for diets such as the Paleo diet mainly because it is very low in calories and is a good source of magnesium and vitamin C that promote healthy digestion and aids in the protection of the body against wounds and viral infections.

• Squash also prevents cancer and most heart ailments plus also promotes proper health of the colon and the prostate, as well. And, if you're having eye problems, you can be sure that by eating squash, your vision will be better and that you can prevent other eye diseases such as glaucoma or catarata from happening. Yep, there's still hope for you!

4. Salmon Eggs Benedict

(Makes 8 servings)

Here's a classy, tasty twist on the breakfast favorite!

Ingredients:

• 2 tsp lemon juice

• 8 eggs

• ¾ cup plain, low-fat yogurt

• 3 egg yolks

• ¼ tsp white sugar

• ¼ tsp salt

• A pinch of ground black pepper

• 8 slices rye bread

• A dash of hot pepper sauce

• 1 Tbsp fresh parsley, chopped

• 8 oz salmon, smoked and cut into small pieces

• 1 tsp capers

Directions:

• Make the sauce by whisking yogurt, egg yolks, lemon juice, salt, mustard, pepper, hot sauce and sugar in a double boiler. Cook for around 6 to 8 minutes or until the mixture evenly simmer.

• Heat 2 quarts of salted water in a stockpot and bring it to a boil. Break the eggs into the pot one at a time, and as gently as you can, and then reduce heat to medium after you have added all the eggs. Remove them with a slotted spoon once they start floating on top.

• Toast bread slices then place them on a serving tray and top each of them with a hot poached egg and a slice of salmon.

• Serve this with a drizzle of yogurt sauce on top. Enjoy!

Health Benefits/Fun Facts:

• Salmon is perfect for you because it contains the best quality of protein and also has a lot of Omega-3 Fatty Acids together with other kinds of vitamins and minerals such as Vitamin A, Vitamin D, Vitamin B and Vitamin E, as well.

• Did you know? April 14th and June 4th are considered as National Eggs Benedict Day!

• Who's Benedict? Well, the name "Benedict" came from a Wall Street Stock Broker named Lemuel Benedict who went to the Waldorf Astoria Hotel in 1894 and who ordered a mix of poached eggs, buttered toast, bacon and hollandaise. The maitre'd was impressed with this dish that he instantly added it to the hotel's menu and named it after Lemuel Benedict! He also substituted bacon with ham and used toasted English muffin instead of buttered toast.

5. Shrimp and Mushroom Quiche

(Makes 8 servings)

Ingredients:

- ½ cup onion, diced
- 1 Tbsp butter
- ½ cup mushrooms, diced
- 2 Tbsp red wine
- ½ tsp fresh parsley, chopped
- 3 eggs
- ¼ tsp red pepper flakes
- ½ cup fat-free sour cream
- 1 cup edam cheese, shredded
- A pinch of salt
- 1 9 inch pie shell (unbaked)
- 1 cup salad shrimp, cooked

Directions:

- Pre-heat the oven to 350 degrees.

- Next, in a skillet, melt butter over medium heat then add the onions and cook until translucent before adding the mushrooms. Cook for 3 minutes more then add the wine and simmer until most of the liquid has evaporated.

- Whisk sour cream, eggs, salt and red pepper flakes in a bowl until smooth then add the cheese. Meanwhile, place the shrimp in the pie shell and sprinkle the mushroom mixture that you have just made on top. Pour the custard and spread it evenly.

• Bake until set or for around 50 minutes then cool for around 10 minutes before serving.

Health Benefits/Fun Facts:

• Losing Weight can be expected once you eat shrimp because it is full of protein, zinc and Vitamin D that can heighten your metabolic levels and certainly make you feel more energetic and in the pink of health. Shrimp also decreases the amount of Leptin in the body. Leptin is the hormone that makes you feel hungry or makes you crave for food, so when you have less of this, you will definitely lose weight!

• Shrimp also contains loads of Anti-oxidants. This means that cells will be regenerated to keep your skin beautiful and young-looking!

• Mushrooms are also known to enhance weight loss. It is said that by eating a cup of mushrooms per day will help someone gain nutrients from meat and yet, will not add in his weight. Mushrooms can also help the body absorb nutrients so that you can be healthy and strong. Plus, mushrooms also enhance the strength of the immune system—making you safe from various diseases, too!

Chapter 2: Let's Have Lunch!

Lunch must be heavy but non-fattening as you're usually out during this time of the day. Lucky for you, here are five Paleo Asian Lunch Recipes that are perfectly suited for those taste buds and that will surely help you get through the day the right way.

6. Cauliflower Thai Rice and Chicken Mix

(Makes 4 servings)

(Asians are known for being lovers of rice and this dish will help you understand why. Forget about rice being bland and all the stuff you've heard—when you do it right, it could be truly flavorful and healthy, too—because you're going to create it from cauliflowers!)

Ingredients:

• 1 Tbsp ginger, freshly grated

• A head of cauliflower

• 3 cloves garlic, crushed

• 3 chilies

• 3 eggs

• Salt, to taste

• 3 to 4 cooked chicken breasts, shredded

• Coconut oil

- ½ cup cilantro, chopped

- 1 Tbsp tamari soy sauce

Directions:

- Break the cauliflower apart into florets then pulse them in a food processor until they resemble the texture and consistency of cooked rice.

- Put the cauliflower in a large pan then cook it with coconut oil. Make sure to stir constantly and to always put the heat on medium only.

- Scramble the eggs in another pan together with some coconut oil then add the cooked eggs to the cauliflower rice.

- Add garlic, chopped chilies and ginger then add the shredded chicken meat once the rice is soft.

- Season with salt and tamari soy sauce and mix thoroughly.

- Garnish with cilantro, if desired then serve and enjoy!

Health Benefits/Fun Facts:

- Cauliflower contains Vitamin K and Omega3 Fatty Acids. It is also full of Manganese and Vitamin C which are both great anti-oxidants. Aside from that, it can also protect you against cardiovascular diseases and cancer, amongst others.

- If you want to detoxify your mind and body and be holistically healthy, cauliflower is the answer to your dilemma. It helps the liver release toxins away from the body so you will feel clean and healthy and ready for whatever life throws at you again.

• Being full of anti-inflammatory properties, cauliflower decreases the risk of diseases such as obesity, ulcer and arthritis and also helps wounds heal fast.

• It also aids in proper digestion, so your metabolic levels can be heightened!

7. Beefy Japanese Curry

(Makes 8 servings)

(This will surely satisfy your spicy craving!)

Ingredients:

• 2 Potatoes

• ½ lb carrots

• 1 Tbsp coconut oil

• 1 medium yellow onion, sliced

• 1 Fuji Apple

• A quart of beef broth

• 1 lb beef, cubed

• 2 garlic cloves, minced

• 2 tsp fresh ginger

• ¼ tsp cayenne pepper

• 2 Tbsp Garam Masala

• 3 Tbsp butter

• 2 Tbsp kosher salt

• 2 tsp curry powder

• 2 Tbsp ketchup

• 2 Tbsp coconut aminos

• 1 ½ Tbsp raw honey

Directions:

• Peel and slice the potatoes into 1 ½ inch thick pieces then soak them in water to remove excess starch. Peel and slice the carrots into 1 inch thick strips as well.

• Next, in a large pot, heat a tablespoon of coconut oil then add onions and cook until translucent. Add garlic and ginger followed by the beef and cook until browned.

• Add salt, carrots, broth and sliced apples then boil for around 20 minutes, uncovered. Make sure to stir constantly then add the potatoes and boil until potatoes are soft or for 15 to 20 minutes more.

• While the potatoes are boiling you should start preparing the curry. To do this, melt the butter in a saucepan then add the tapioca starch and whisk them together thoroughly. Heat for around 15 to 20 minutes while whisking occasionally then remove from heat and add the curry powder, cayenne pepper and garam masala.

• Ladle around half a cup of the stew broth and mix it with the curry. Add ketchup, coconut aminos and honey together with the rest of the broth.

• Season to taste then serve with rice or cauliflower rice, if desired. Enjoy!

Health Benefits/Fun Facts:

• Did you know? Curry actually comes from the Tamil word "kari", which means "sautéed vegetables" or "spices".

• London has the most number of curry restaurants in the world! Its first curry restaurant opened in 1810 and is called "Shayk Din Mahomet".

• In 1846, a poem entitled "A Poem to Curry" was published as part of the book "Kitchen Melodies" by William Makepeace Thackeray.

• Garam Masala is considered as the "magic spice" because it is a blend of most ground spices that can be used especially for Asian Dishes to give them a distinct flair.

• Carrots are popular for being good for one's vision but aside from that, it's also great in preventing cancer, especially breast and colon cancer, and is also full of anti-oxidants that promote glowing, healthy skin. This is why carrots are known for their beautifying and anti-aging properties! Aside from that, carrots also prevent heart diseases and strokes and also promote healthy teeth and gums. They also detoxify the body and rid it of toxins.

8. Filipino Style Roasted Chicken with Veggies

(Makes 4 servings)

(More often than not, when there are festivities and gatherings in the Philippines, roasted chicken is served. The delicious aroma makes people nostalgic about their childhood and makes them want to eat—fast!)

Ingredients:

• One 5 to 6 lb roasting chicken

• A large bunch of fresh thyme

• Freshly ground black pepper

• Kosher salt

• 1 head garlic, cut in half

• 1 lemon, cut in half

• 4 carrots, cut into chunks

• 1 large yellow onion, sliced thickly

• 2 Tbsp butter

• 1 fennel bulb, tops removed then cut into wedges

• Olive oil

• Brussels sprouts, to taste

Directions:

• Pre-heat the oven to 425 degrees.

• Rinse the chicken thoroughly and trim off any excess fat. Pat it dry and liberally season with salt and pepper.

• Stuff the chicken with the lemon, garlic, and half a bunch of thyme then brush the outside with butter.

• Tie the legs with some kitchen string and tuck its wings under its body and put it on top of the onions, carrots and fennel in the roasting pan.

• Toss extra thyme, salt, pepper and olive oil together with the rest of the ingredients and spread the mixture evenly to the bottom of the pan before placing the chicken on top.

• Proceed to roasting the chicken for an hour and a half or until the juices have run clear then move the chicken and the vegetables to another platter and cover for around 20 minutes with aluminum foil.

• Slice the chicken before serving and serve with vegetables on the side. Enjoy!

Health Benefits/Fun Facts:

• What's good about chicken is that it is full of protein that promotes muscle growth instead of fats. It is also a natural anti-depressant—that's why parents/guardians usually make chicken soup when a child is not feeling well. It's because chicken increases the body's happy hormones or the Serotonin levels in the brain to keep a person feeling calm and good.

• Chicken also prevents bone damage and bone loss—so even if you're no longer young, you can expect that you can still live a happy, adventurous life!

• Meanwhile, thyme protects the body's cell membranes and is also a very powerful anti-oxidant. It also protects the body against microbes and is a good source of Vitamin C, as well—so it can protect you against the common colds, coughs and flu!

• Kosher Salt is healthy for you because it contains no additives and can regulate muscle growth and contractions because of its high vitamin and mineral content.

9. Paleo Caldereta (Beef and Veggie Stew)

(Makes 6 servings)

(Caldereta is one of the well-loved Filipino dishes of all time and this one is the healthy, non-fattening version!)

Ingredients:

- 1 onion, diced

- 2 lbs grass-fed beef, cubed

- 1 tomato, diced

- 5 oz grass-fed liverwurst

- 1 Tbsp red chili flakes, dried

- 5 garlic cloves, minced

- ½ cups carrot discs

- 2 cups beef broth

- 1 can tomato paste

- 1 can tomato sauce

- 2 Tbsp rice vinegar

- 3 bay leaves

- 2 cups green beans, sliced

- 1 orange pepper, sliced

- 1 red pepper, sliced

- 2 Tbsp lard

- 1 Tbsp paprika

- ½ cup coconut aminos

- Salt and pepper, to taste

Directions:

- Pre-heat oven to 325 degrees then place liverwurst, tomato paste and tomato sauce in a blender or food processor and puree them and season the beef with salt and pepper.

- Next, add a tablespoon of lard to a Dutch oven then sauté onions, carrots, garlic and chili pepper flakes until translucent. Turn the heat to low after adding chopped tomatoes then simmer for a minute or two before turning the heat off.

- Then, heat a skillet then add the other tablespoon of lard before adding the seasoned beef. Cook until browned then transfer to the Dutch oven.

- Mix coconut aminos with vinegar in a glass then pour over the beef bits to deglaze them. Move everything to the Dutch oven then add the pureed tomato paste, tomato sauce and liverwurst together with paprika, beef broth and bay leaves to the oven and mix thoroughly.

- Bake the mixture for around an hour then add the green beans and bake for 20 minutes more. Then, add the bell peppers and bake again for 10 minutes.

- Serve with steamed cauliflower rice, if desired. Enjoy!

Health Benefits/Fun Facts:

• The usual Caldereta is historically made with goat shoulders with liver spread and tomato paste. It is well-loved for its spicy flavor.

• Because it is spicy, Caldereta is full of Capsaicin. This means that it enhances the body's metabolic levels so food can easily be digested and so you would not get fat easily.

• Caldereta is usually served during different kinds of festivities and parties, especially during a town "fiesta" or the feast of a Patron Saint.

• Instead of using soy sauce that's full of sodium, you can opt for coconut aminos instead. They have low acid content and are certified to be raw and gluten-free and is also low in glycemic index because of its sap.

10. Chinese Orange Chicken

(Makes 6 servings)

(Orange Chicken is a traditional Chinese favorite. What makes this recipe special is that it is made with Sriracha, or a sauce made out of chili peppers so it has this distinct flair that will set it apart from the rest!)

Ingredients:

- 3 ½ lb chicken or 10 chicken drumsticks

- 2 tsp kosher salt

- **For the marinade**: 1 cup fresh basil leaves, packed

- 1 medium yellow onion, chopped roughly

- 4 garlic cloves, chopped roughly

- ½ cup orange juice

- 1 tsp tomato paste

- 1 Tbsp balsamic vinegar

- 1 Tbsp fish sauce

- ½ tsp freshly ground black pepper

- **For the Orange Sriracha Sauce:** 2 Tbsp honey

- ½ cup orange juice

- 1 Tbsp ghee

- 1 Tbsp Paleo Sriracha

- 1 tsp sesame seeds, toasted

- 1 tsp coconut aminos

- Kosher salt

Directions:

- Place the chicken on a bowl and sprinkle salt all over it. Make the marinade by tossing basil, onion, garlic, orange juice, balsamic vinegar, fish sauce, pepper and tomato paste altogether in a blender or a food processor. Puree the ingredients until smooth.

- Pour the said mixture over the chicken then cover the chicken and marinade it for an hour to a full 12 hours.

- Once the chicken is ready to cook, place the pieces on a wire rack then spoon marinade over each piece of chicken and bake until cooked through or for around 40 minutes. Make sure to flip each piece halfway through then make the sriracha sauce while the chicken is baking.

- Mix all of the sriracha ingredients together in a small bowl then cook it for around 3 to 5 minutes in high heat. Season to taste.

- After roasting the chicken for 40 minutes, spread Sriracha sauce all over them then roast them for 5 minutes more. Take the tray out of the oven and glaze the chicken with the rest of the sauce.

- Serve with sesame seeds on top and enjoy!

Health Benefits/Fun Facts:

- The recipe for Orange Chicken originally came from the Hunan Cuisine of China or from people who live near the Xiang River. Most of their dishes are popular for their deep color and fresh aroma and the fact that their flavors are more often than not, spicy and hot!

• Meanwhile, Balsamic Vinegar is extremely beneficial because it reduces the risk of certain diseases such as Cancer and heart problems and is also a very powerful anti-oxidant for it destroys free radicals in the body. Free radicals are elements that destroy cell membranes so you definitely do not need them!

• Balsamic Vinegar also promotes better digestion and is a great pain reliever, and also aids in weight loss, as well.

Chapter 3: What's for Dinner?

Dinner is usually where the magic happens. It's a time for celebration and for having fun whether by yourself or with the people you love. And that's why you should always prepare sumptuous meals during this time of the day. It's also important to make sure that what you prepare for dinner is light but enticing—and these dishes below perfect sum it all up.

11. Japanese Lemon and Garlic Shrimp

(Makes 4 to 6 servings)

(This is usually served at parties, especially engagement parties for it's just light but truly filling!)

Ingredients:

- ½ fresh lemon juice

- 1 lb shrimp, deveined

- 3 Tbsp organic, grass-fed ghee

- 3 to 4 cloves garlic, chopped

- 1 Tbsp fresh parsley, chopped

- Freshly ground pepper, to taste

Directions:

- Heat the pan to medium heat then add garlic and ghee and sauté for at least a minute.

• Add the shrimp then sauté each side for a minute.

• Add lemon juice, Himalayan salt and pepper then sauté for a minute more then take it off from the heat and place in a bowl or a plate.

• Serve with fresh parsley, if desired.

• Enjoy!

Health Benefits/Fun Facts:

• Lemons alkalize the body. This means that they decrease the acidic levels in the body and only retain what's proper.

• Lemons are also important in detoxifying the liver and are rich in flavonoids or vitamin C that protects the body against coughs and colds. Lemons are also said to help in the treatment of scurvy, also known as the bleeding gum disease and can also destroy intestinal worms.

• In Ayurveda, lemons are beneficial because they promote good vision and light.

• Garlic is high in iodine so it can protect you against goiter plus it also helps babies grow while they are still in the womb.

• There are certain folklores in Asia that say that garlic can protect someone against vampires and evil spirits—and that's why some people hang a bunch of garlic on their door!

12. Shabu-Shabu Paleo Platter

(Makes 2 servings)

(This is a perfect party dish that's light but still filling!)

Ingredients:

• ½ shabu-shabu grass-fed beef, sliced thinly

• A large pot of chicken or bone broth

• Radishes, spinach, sweet potato or any other vegetable of your choice

• Gluten-free tamari sauce

Directions:

• In a large pot, boil the broth then add the meat and vegetables in.

• Boil the contents of the pot until the meat is browned and until the vegetables are soft.

• Serve this dish with gluten-free tamari sauce and enjoy!

Health Benefits/Fun Facts:

• Shabu-Shabu is basically a dish made out of thin beef slices that are boiled in water. It was introduced in Japan during the 20th century when a restaurant called "Suehiro" opened. If you're ever going to visit Tokyo or any other tourist hot spots in Japan, you can expect that you'll easily find Shabu-Shabu.

• The name "Shabu-Shabu" was coined because of the sound that the meat emits when it is being cooked.

• Some people are also fond of using top sirloin, crab meat, pork, lamb, chicken, or duck in their Shabu-Shabus.

13. Amazing Almond Pork

(Makes 2 to 4 servings)

(This is a Thai delicacy that is truly sumptuous. The blend of pork and almond butter is just to-die-for!)

Ingredients:

- 1 ½ Tbsp coconut oil

- 1 ¼ lbs sliced grass-fed pork tenderloin

- 5 Thai chilies, chopped

- 3 Tbsp almond butter

- 2 bell peppers, sliced

- 2 cups broccoli florets

- 3 tsp sesame oil

- 1 tsp fish sauce

- ½ cup coconut milk

- 2 pinches of sea salt

- 1 tsp grated ginger

Directions:

• To prepare the sauce, mix the Thai chilies, almond butter, sesame oil, fish sauce and coconut milk in a small bowl until well-blended then mix bell peppers and broccoli in a small wok together with ¼ cup of water. Cook for around 6 to 8 minutes in medium heat.

• Cook ginger, green onions and coconut oil in a skillet over medium heat for 3 minutes then add the sliced pork and cook until both sides are brown or for 3 to 5 minutes. Make sure not to overcook then add the ingredients from the skillet to the wok before adding the almond sauce. Cover for around 10 minutes and simmer on low.

Health Benefits/Fun Facts:

• Did you know? Almonds actually came from the family of Peaches! That's why sometimes they are called as "stone fruits" instead of nuts.

• Speaking of still being nuts, almonds are cool because they have the lowest calorie content and can be eaten whether raw or roasted. It's also easy to create your own almond butter or almond milk that you can use for various recipes such as the one above.

• Broccoli was first planted in the Mediterranean Isles in the 6th century. It's quite beneficial because it contains high Vitamin C content. In fact, a cup of broccoli is already equivalent to the Vitamin C content of one orange!

• Broccoli is also very high in fiber and is also anti-inflammatory. It protects the body against various diseases, especially against heart ailments and bronchitis.

• California produces the most number of broccolis in the United States and that's why it is sometimes called as the "Broccoli Nation".

14. Duck Paleo Okonomiyaki

(Makes 4 servings)

(Okonomiyaki is commonly known as a Pizza Pancake in Japan and is usually served during celebrations or gatherings so if you're having any dinner parties, you should definitely try making this one!)

Ingredients:

- **For the Duck:** ½ tsp five spice powder

- 2 duck breasts (skin intact)

- Salt and pepper, to taste

- **For Okonomiyaki:** ½ cup bean sprouts

- ½ cup Napa cabbage, sliced

- 2 Tbsp fennel leaves

- 3 green onion stalks

- ¾ cup chicken stock

- 3 eggs

- 3 Tbsp coconut flour

- 3 Tbsp Tapioca Starch

- Vegetable oil

- ¼ cup shitake mushrooms, sliced

- 1 tsp garlic, chopped

- ¼ cup carrots, shredded

Directions:

• Pre-heat oven to 375 degrees. Score the skin of the duck in a criss-cross pattern. Make sure not to slice into the meat.

• Put the duck breasts on a skillet on a medium-high heat, skin side down then cook for around 10 minutes, covered, before transferring the duck to a shallow pan. Once in the shallow pan, roast the duck for around 10 to 15 minutes in the oven until temperature reaches 155 degrees.

• Let the duck sit and start preparing the Okonomiyaki. To do this, sift the coconut flour with the tapioca starch then whisk the chicken stock in and allow sitting for another minute.

• Mix the eggs in and blend using a hand mixer or a food processor.

• Add the carrots, cabbage, sprouts and fennel and fold them all in. Heat the skillet with a tablespoon of oil again then pour around half a cup of the mixture in.

• Cook for around 4 minutes while covered with parchment paper then flip it up and cook for 3 to 4 minutes more.

• Serve with your choice of Paleo Mayonnaise or Okonomiyaki Sauce made with Sake, molasses and tomato paste. To do make your own okonomiyaki sauce, just mix Worcestershire sauce, vinegar, tomato paste, raw honey, blackstrap molasses, allspice, coconut aminos, sake and white wine altogether.

• To make Paleo Mayo, simply combine vinegar, eggs, salt, mustard and cayenne pepper in a food processor or blender then pulse until frothy. While pulsing, add some extra virgin olive oil until the mixture emulsifies then add the rest of the oil and add salt, as well. You may keep this in the fridge for around a week if covered tightly.

• You may also serve the okonomiyaki with sliced shitake mushrooms.

• Serve and enjoy!

Health Benefits/Fun Facts:

• Okonomiyaki literally means "Grilled as you like it".

• Before the Second World War, Okonomiyaki was invented in Japan and became popular during the war and even after. A sweeter version is called as the "Sukesoyaki" and is often served at Buddhist ceremonies.

• It is said that serving Okonomiyaki with mayonnaise was started by a restaurant in 1946.

• Kansai and Hiroshima are two of the most popular types of Okonomiyaki. Kansai is made with batter that is made of bonito flakes and flour mixed with yam and dried leaves while Hiroshima is basically Okonomiyaki that is layered instead of being mixed together. Hiroshima style is also sweeter than Kansai.

15. Cod and Calamari Surprise

(Makes 2 to 4 servings)

Ingredients:

- ½ lb cod, cut into ½ inch thick pieces

- 2 cups calamari tentacles

- 2 Tbsp ghee

- 1 large white onion

- 1 red bell pepper

- 1 green bell pepper

- ¼ cup water

- 1 can coconut milk

- 3 dried Thai chilies

- ½ inch grated fresh ginger root

- 1 ½ cup dried Porcini mushrooms

- 2 Tbsp fish sauce

- 1 tsp black sesame seeds

- ¼ tsp cayenne

- ¼ tsp coconut sugar

- 1/3 Tbsp five spice powder

Directions:

• Soak the Porcini mushrooms in a small bowl for around 10 minutes then drain. After draining, sauté the mushrooms with the other vegetables.

• Heat the ghee on a large pan on high heat then add the dried Thai chilies and sliced onions and stir-fry until golden brown. Add five spice powder and the sliced bell peppers together with fish sauce, black sesame seeds, cayenne, coconut sugar, fresh ginger root, and the sautéed mushrooms and then cook in medium high for around 5 minutes then add water and coconut milk. Stir constantly.

• After reducing heat to low, add the cod and calamari tentacles and simmer for another 10 to 15 minutes more and serve with cauliflower rice.

• Enjoy!

Health Benefits/Fun Facts:

• In many restaurants all over Asia, fried calamari is a popular appetizer because it's delectable and easy to eat.

• Calamari is actually quite low in fat and calories. Actually, it only has 26 calories per ounce! It is also a good source of protein, so you can be sure that it is healthy and right for you.

• Meanwhile, cod is considered as one of the healthiest fish in the world because it increases the heart's vitality because of its Omega 3 content. It protects the heart against fatal diseases such as Arrythmia and can also lower the fat and cholesterol content of the body. Aside from that, it also controls and prevents high blood pressure and thrombosis, as well.

Chapter 4: Snack Time is Fun

When it comes to snacks, you have to be careful and not rely on the usual junk food or chips that you once enjoyed when you were young. You can create an entirely new breed of Paleo Asian-inspired snacks that will give a whole new meaning to the word "snacks".

16. Pork Aloha Skewers

(Makes 4 to 8 servings)

(Asians, especially Filipinos love adding pineapples on various dishes. This is one perfect example that you absolutely have to try as it's perfect for bonding with the ones you love, especially on birthday parties and the like!)

Ingredients:

• **For the skewers:** 1 lb pork chops, boneless and center-cut into 1 inch cubes

• 1 bell pepper, cut into chunks

• Fresh pineapple chunks

• Red cocktail onions

• **For the marinade:** 2 Tbsp rice wine vinegar

• 4 Tbsp coconut aminos

• 2 Tbsp sesame seeds

• 1 Tbsp sesame oil, toasted

- 1 tsp freshly grated ginger

- 1 tsp red pepper flakes, crushed

- 1 tsp fresh garlic, chopped

- 1 Tbsp black pepper

Directions:

• Make the marinade first by mixing together all of the ingredients for the marinade together with the pork. Refrigerate for around 4 hours or overnight for flavors to be well-infused. Soak the skewers in water for around 30 minutes to make sure that they do not burn.

• Place pork, onion, pineapple and peppers onto the skewers alternately then grill the skewers on high heat until pork is cooked through.

Health Benefits/Fun Facts:

• Skewers are called "espentihos" in Portuguese and "brochettes" in French. You can mix and match your own ingredients. The most popular ones include meat, seafood and fruits.

• Pineapples actually originated in Europe and not in Hawaii!

• Pineapples are also beneficial because they protect you against high blood pressure, Asthma, macular degeneration, diabetes and cancer. They also aid in fertility and aids in proper healing of wounds because of its anti-inflammatory properties. The said fruit can also protect you against kidney stones and is very high in fiber so it can rid the body of toxins—making you feel healthy and clean all at once.

17. The Best Green Papaya Salad

(Makes 2 servings)

Ingredients:

- ½ cucumber

- 4 cups shredded green papaya

- ¼ cup fresh lime juice

- ½ cup Thai Basil leaves, washed and packed

- 1 to 2 Red Thai Chili Peppers

- 12 green beans

- 3 green onions

- 2 Tbsp dried shrimp

- 1 Tbsp coconut aminos

- 2 Tbsp fish sauce

Directions:

• Peel the papaya, and using a sharp knife, cut it into julienned pieces then prepare the rest of the vegetables.

• Slice the cucumber lengthwise after peeling then scoop out the seeds then chop the cherry tomatoes into quarters and slice the onions into small pieces that resemble matchsticks and slice the green beans, as well. Chop the basil leaves roughly and mix all the vegetables together with the papaya in a bowl.

• Pour the juice of the limes over the vegetables then add coconut aminos and fish sauce with a drizzle of honey, then add the dried shrimp and let the mixture sit until all the flavors have been incorporated or for around 30 minutes.

• Garnish the salad with cilantro and chopped cashews then serve and enjoy! This is the perfect snack to eat after eating a beef or fish dish.

Health Benefits/Fun Facts:

• Green Papaya Salad is known as "Atchara" in the Philippines and "Som Tam" in Thailand. It is known for its tart and spicy flavor.

• Papaya is a great fruit because it is the perfect cure for menstrual pain. So, if you're a woman and you hate having those monthly woes and sickness, you can try eating papaya and see the good benefits for yourself.

• Papaya is also known to heal the body's skin problems and wounds and can regulate bowel moments. Aside from that, it also burns fat and calories so you can be sure that you'll be able to lose weight fast and in the natural manner.

18. Chicken Patties served with Cabbage Slaw

(Makes 2 to 4 servings)

Ingredients:

• **For the Patties:** ½ cup green onions, sliced diagonally

• 1 lb ground chicken/turkey

• 1 Tbsp coconut aminos

• 2 Tbsp dark sesame oil

• ¼ cup cilantro, chopped finely

• 2 to 3 garlic cloves, minced

• 2 Tbsp fresh ginger, grated

• 1 large egg

• 1 to 2 squirts of Sriracha

• **For the Cabbage Slaw:** zest of 1 lime

• 4 cups of white and purple cabbage, sliced thinly

• 1 Jalapeno pepper, seeded and minced

• ¼ cup cilantro, chopped

• 1 Tbsp dark sesame oil

• ½ tsp sea salt

• 1 to 2 Tbsp lime juice, freshly squeezed

• 2 ripe avocados

• 1 tsp honey, warmed

Directions:

• Make the slaw first by mixing all of the ingredients together except the avocado. Chill this for around 15 minutes or up to an hour.

• To make the patties, break the ground meat into small pieces in a large bowl then add all of the ingredients. Mix them thoroughly with your hands then make around 4 to 8 patties out of the meat.

• Place the patties on a lined cookie sheet then freeze for around 5 minutes. This will make the patties firm.

• Heat a tablespoon of coconut oil over medium heat in the stove then add the patties to the pan. Fry each side for 3 to 4 minutes then serve with the prepared cabbage slaw and Sriracha sauce.

• Garnish with cilantro and enjoy!

Health Benefits/Fun Facts:

• While most people just disregard cabbage, it is actually one of the best vegetables for weight loss and is also considered as a food for the brain because it heightens stimuli and helps the brain process things easily, as well.

• Cabbage is also considered as a beautifying mineral because it is high in sulfur and can prevent blood pressure from getting high. It also regulates the blood sugar so diabetes and heart problems can be prevented and is also beneficial against headaches.

19. Salted Duck Egg Yolks with French Beans

(Makes 3 servings)

Ingredients:

• 3 pcs salted duck egg yolks

• 300 grams French Beans

• Salt

• Oil

• 1 garlic clove, crushed

Directions:

• Boil the duck eggs first then separate the whites from the yolks after cooking. Mash the yolks and set the whites aside.

• Mix the garlic with oil and French beans in a wok and fry until thoroughly cooked.

• Add the yolks and toss until well-combined. Before serving, season with salt and enjoy!

Health Benefits/Fun Facts:

• Salted eggs are rich in amino acids, calcium, protein, phosphorus and iron. It basically contains everything you need for your body to grow sturdy and healthy.

• Meanwhile, French Beans only contain 31 calories per bunch so they are definitely great for weight loss. Aside from that, they are also rich in dietary fiber which the body needs to be able to live a healthy and well-balanced life.

• The Vitamin A content of French Beans promote proper and healthy vision and are also full of anti-oxidants that get rid of free radicals in the body.

• French Beans are also beneficial for pregnant and lactating women because of their high folate content. They also protect the body against microbes and prevent various diseases from happening.

20. Steak Lettuce Wraps with Quick Pickles

(Makes 2 to 4 servings)

(If you're looking for a snack that will fill you up but is still filled with all the nutrients you need, you should definitely try this one!)

Ingredients:

• Bibb lettuce cups

• 1 lb flank steak

• 1 to ½ knob fresh ginger, peeled and chopped

• 1 to 1 ½ Tbsp creamy almond butter

• 2 garlic cloves

• ½ Tbsp red chili pepper flakes

• 1 Tbsp + 1 tsp sesame oil

• 2 Tbsp honey

• 3 Tbsp extra virgin olive oil

• 3 Tbsp fresh lime juice

• ¼ cup soy sauce

For the Quick Pickles:

• 1 small red onion, sliced thinly

• 1 small cucumber, peeled and sliced thinly

• 2 tsp sugar

• ¼ cup rice vinegar

Directions:

• To make the quick pickles, just mix all of the Quick Pickle ingredients together in a bowl. Stir until well-combined and set aside in the refrigerator. You can make this a day before serving, if desired

• Next, combine lime juice, soy sauce, honey, olive oil, red chili pepper flakes, garlic, ginger and sesame oil in a food processor or blender and pulse until smooth. Take out at least ¼ cup of the liquid and then mix it with almond butter in the blender. Process the mixture again until smooth.

• Add the rest of the marinade to the steak and marinade for around 10 to 15 minutes on the counter.

• Then, pre-heat a grill pan to high heat and cook the steak until medium rare. Move the steak to a cutting board and slice against the grain after cooling for 10 minutes.

• Serve the steak on the lettuce cups together with the quick pickle mix and with a drizzle of almond butter sauce on top.

Health Benefits/Fun Facts:

• Flank Steak contains a lot of fiber and that's why most gym buffs and body-builders choose it over other kinds of meat. It's also rich in protein and contains a low amount of calories, too.

• Meanwhile, cucumber is said to boost the body's happy hormones and can also rehydrate and replenish the body with water. It's also good for hair and skin care and relieved the body of bad breath—so you should definitely eat cucumbers before going out on a date!

• Cucumbers also promote proper digestion so they're beneficial when it comes to weight loss. They also contain loads of anti-oxidants and that's why they are used for most beauty regimens. Aside from that, cucumbers also promote proper joint health and protect the body against arthritis and gout, too. If you are already experiencing gout, you can eat cucumbers to relieve the pain that you are feeling.

Chapter 5: Sweet Dessert Treats

Just because you're following a healthy diet regimen doesn't mean that you can no longer try sweet treats. After reading this chapter, you'll certainly be able to make amazing Paleo Asian Desserts that will be the talk of the town for ages!

21. Awesome ABC (Ais Batu Campur)/Colorful Shaved Ice Treat

(Makes 1 to 2 servings)

(This Malaysian treat is probably one of the most interesting desserts you'll ever taste. It is made of shaved ice and topped with different kinds of colorful beans, which makes it interesting and truly delicious!)

Ingredients:

• **For the ABC:** evaporated milk

• Ice, shaved finely

• Red beans, cooked

• Rose syrup

• Palm sugar syrup

• **For the toppings:** Durian Ice cream

• 75 grams jelly

• 1 tin of creamy sweet corn

- Bananas, sliced

- 45 grams palm seed

- 80 grams roasted peanuts, crushed finely

Directions:

- To cook the red beans, rinse them in running water and let them soak for around 2 hours, and then put the beans in a pot of water with Pandan leaves. Boil water on low-medium heat then lower the heat once the beans are soft. Make sure to stir this regularly and to add sugar until the beans are mushy. Allow the beans to cool after removing from heat.

- To cook the palm syrup, mix the Pandan leaves and palm sugar together with water in a pot then boil the water. Once the syrup is thick, lower the heat then remove from heat after allowing the syrup to cool down.

- Now, to make and arrange the ABC, just put some finely shaved ice in a bowl then infuse it with flavors by adding palm sugar syrup, evaporated milk and rose syrup. Top it with red beans, peanuts and sweet corn. You may also layer these toppings with ice then top it again with whatever you have left.

- Serve this dessert with a topping of durian ice cream and enjoy!

Health Benefits/Fun Facts:

- In the Philippines, "Ais Batu Campur" is called as Halo-Halo and is usually served during the summer season to beat the heat.

- Red Beans are full of fiber, iron and protein. Because of this, you can be sure that digestive processes will be regulated and that your body will produce muscles instead of fat. Also, red beans are considered as one of those foods that are high in anti-oxidants so if you're concerned about the state of your hair and skin, you can try eating these beans.

• Durian is very popular in Asia, especially in the province of Davao in the Philippines for its pungent smell. However, once you try it and once you try delicacies such as candies, pastries and ice cream made out of it, you'll understand why so many people love it!

• The name "Durian" comes from the Malay word "Duri", which means "thorn".

• Sweet corn is gluten-free and can be used for Paleo/Gluten-free meals and by people who are affected by the celiac disease. It is also one of the best sources of dietary fiber, ferulic acid and anti-oxidants, as well.

• And the best thing about sweet corn is that it contains all of the Vitamin B Complex nutrients that you need for the body's metabolic levels to be heightened.

22. Sticky Rice and Mango

(Makes 6 servings)

(This is a traditional Thai dessert that's sure to satisfy your sweet tooth!)

Ingredients:

• 250 ml coconut milk

• 400 grams Thai rice

• 6 ripe yellow mangoes

• 1 tsp salt

• 100 grams white sugar

• 2 Tbsp sesame seeds, toasted

Directions:

• Submerge the sticky rice in water and let it soak for 5 to 8 hours or overnight then drain it in a steamer and steam until the rice is well-done.

• Put three tablespoons of coconut milk in a pot then cook it until it is hot. Set the coconut milk aside.

• Mix sugar, salt and the remaining coconut milk in a bowl until both the salt and sugar are dissolved then add the sticky rice that you have steamed and add the coconut milk, as well. Let the mixture stand for around 15 minutes, covered.

• Remove the pits of the mango off its skin then slice it into strips and serve on a platter.

• Scoop the rice into the mango platter once it is cool then sprinkle sesame seeds and coconut milk on top.

• Serve immediately and enjoy!

Health Benefits/Fun Facts:

• In India, Mangoes are known as "safeda".

• Mangoes are beneficial because they lower the cholesterol levels, they clear the skin and eliminate clogged pores, and some health experts also say that they can prevent cancer.

• Just like carrots, mangoes are also great for the eyes as they promote better vision and better eye health. A cup of mangoes can already provide the body with 25% of its daily Vitamin A need that can prevent dry eyes and blindness, too. Mangoes also alkalize the body because of its citric and tartaric acid content.

• And, guess what? Mangoes are great against heat stroke—they can rehydrate the body easily plus they also improve digestion and promote a healthy sex life, too! And more than that, they are great for strengthening the immune system and helping you live a healthier, well-balanced life.

• In the Philippines, there is a gelatinous/sticky rice dessert called "Suman" which is usually served with coconut jam or sugar! Yummy!

23. Milky Melon with Sago

(Makes 5 servings)

Ingredients:

• 1 cup sago (aka Tapioca Pearls)

• 1 small honeydew melon

• 1 cup coconut milk (canned if you cannot find fresh) mixed with a teaspoon of salt

• ½ cup water

• ½ cup sugar

Directions:

• In a medium-sized pot, boil water and sugar together. When the sugar is fully dissolved and the mixture attains a syrupy texture, take off the heat and set aside.

• In a separate pot, bring to a boil around 7 cups of water and add the tapioca pearls. Cook the pearls on medium-high until they become translucent. Make sure not to overcook because the tapioca pearls will dissolve. Stir constantly to avoid the tapioca pearls from sticking to the pot.

• Once the pearls are cooked, use a sieve to drain it under running water before setting it aside.

• Scoop out the flesh of the melon (or cantaloupe) using a melon baller. You may also choose to just dice the melon, if desired.

• Set aside one half of the melons then use a food processor to blend the rest of the fruit.

• Mix the melon, sago, and coconut milk together in a bowl; make sure to chill it before serving.

Health Benefits/Fun Facts:

• Melon has high water content—so they're definitely beneficial for rehydrating the body and ridding it of toxins.

• Melon is also good for the heart. In fact, it can protect the body against most heart diseases because of its carotenoid content that also prevents cancer from happening, as well.

• If you want healthy and beautiful skin, you should go on and eat melons because they have high collagen content that makes the skin look divine and lovely. It also works for healing wounds and can cure eczema and kidney diseases. Aside from that, melon also gets rid of heartburn so proper digestion is promoted and pain can be alleviated.

• Sago or Tapioca Pearls actually come from the Sago Palm. It can be propagated by seeds and it's so easy to care for the tree where it comes from.

• In some Asian countries, sago is added in drinks or coolers and is patronized by everyone from young to old!

• And while it's called "Sago Palm", it is actually not a "palm" but a tree that has been on earth for over 200 million years now. Wow!

24. Awesome Pandan Kaya Cake

(Makes 3 to 4 servings)

Ingredients:

• 4 eggs

• 250 grams Paleo Sponge Cake Flour Mix

• Green Pandan Paste

• 3 Tbsp Pandan Juice

• 1 ½ Tbsp corn oil

• 3 Tbsp thick coconut milk

• **For the Pandan Kaya (Caramelized Pandan Sauce):** 9 Tbsp green pea flour

• 180 grams sugar

• 1 Tbsp instant jelly powder

• Pandan paste

• Green coloring

• ½ tsp salt

• 60 grams desiccated coconut

Directions:

• To make the cake, whisk the eggs with flour until light and fluffy then add some Pandan juice and whisk some more.

• Add pandan paste and green coloring then add corn oil and coconut milk and fold until well-combined.

• Pour the mixture into a 9 inch round cake pan and bake for around 40 to 45 minutes at 175 degrees.

• Slice the cake on a wire rack and let cool for a bit.

• To make the Pandan Kaya, just put all of the Kaya ingredients in a pot and mix them all thoroughly. Cook until the mixture is smooth and thick then place a slice of the cake into a cake ring and pour a bit of the Pandan Kaya sauce in. Repeat the process until you are able to cover the rest of the cake with Pandan Kaya.

• Let the cake chill in the fridge then remove the cake from the ring and sprinkle desiccated coconut on top.

• Slice the cake and make sure to serve it chilled. Enjoy!

Health Benefits/Fun Facts:

• Pandan is quite popular in Asian countries because of its aroma and the fact that it makes people want to eat.

• Pandan is beneficial because it reduces fever, relieves the pain from arthritis and headaches, treats ear infections and chest pains, and can also be the cure for leprosy, small pox and certain kinds of wounds. Aside from that, it is also popular for being able to cure skin problems and make the skin healthy and more beautiful plus it also does wonders for women who have just given birth because it hastens the healing process and make women ready for life again!

• Coconuts are rich in fiber and Vitamin C. Not only will it help in detoxifying your body, it can also help in regulating your bowel movement and in making sure that your body gets to absorb all the nutrients it needs easily, too!

• Coconut milk is also perfect for people who are lactose intolerant. If you have been plagued with not being able to drink milk your whole life, now's your chance to do so with the help of coconut milk!

25. Jelly Mountain Paradise

(Makes 2 to 3 servings)

(This amazing Asian dessert was created as a tribute to Kota Kinabalu, an island in Malaysia that is popular for being one of the world's hidden paradises. It has four layers, one being the sky, followed by the mountain, the grass and finally, the land. You'll certainly have fun creating this one! It is also a feast for the eyes.)

Ingredients:

• **For the mountain:** 1 tsp caster sugar

• 50 ml water

• Juice from 3 to 4 bunga telang (blue pea flower, a flowering plant)

• ¼ tsp agar powder

• **For the sky:** 2 Tbsp fresh and thick coconut milk

• ¼ tsp agar powder

• 50 ml water

• Juice from 2 bunga telang

• 1 tsp caster sugar

• **For the grass:** 1 small Pandan leaf, massage with ½ cup water and pounded

• 100 ml water

• ½ tsp agar powder

• 2 tsp caster sugar

- **For the land**: 2 cups water

- 3 Tbsp white pearl sago

- 2 Tbsp Gula Melaka syrup

Directions:

- Make the mountain first by mixing the agar powder and sugar together and sprinkle it over the water. Heat gently until sugar is dissolved and then mix with the bunga telang juice. Stir thoroughly.

- Pour the liquidized agar in a mold through a sieve then set aside.

- To make the sky, mix sugar and agar powder again in a bowl and sprinkle it over the water. Heat until sugar is dissolved and then mix with the bunga telang juice. Stir well. Pour the mixture again in a mold and set aside after sieving on top of the mountain.

- To make the grass, mix sugar and agar powder together and sprinkle the mixture over water in a pot. Heat until sugar is dissolved. Remove the mixture from heat. Mix with pandan water and stir constantly.

- Sieve it over the sky and keep them chilled.

- To make the land, add white sago pearls in a pot of boiling water then stir constantly to make sure that the pearls do not stick to the pot. Boil gently until pearls are transparent then turn off heat after covering. If the center of the pearls are still white after around 10 minutes, turn back the heat and repeat this process.

- Pour the pearls through a sieve in running water so starch will be removed. Use a spoon to stir until all excess water and pearls are gone.

• Add gula Melaka and mix thoroughly and scoop this over the green layer. Chill for around 8 to 9 hours, covered.

• Serve the Jelly Paradise with Gula Melaka and fresh coconut milk. Enjoy!

Health Benefits/Fun Facts:

• Gula Melaka is a term used for sago/tapioca pearls with sugar. Sometimes, it is also called as "sago pudding".

• Bunga Telang or Blue Pea Flower is used as a natural food dye for making various Asian Sweets. It comes from the Blue Pea Flower Plant that blooms in just a matter of 6 weeks! It's also very useful since you can use it for a long time once kept in a cool, dry place.

Conclusion

Thank you again for downloading this book!

I hope you enjoyed reading about my book on 25 Paleo Asian Recipes!

Finally, if you enjoyed this book, please take the time to share your thoughts and **post a review**. It'd be greatly appreciated!

Thank you!